DIABETIC COOKBOOK

50 INTRODUCTORY RECIPES TO GET YOU STARTED IN MANAGING DIABETES

Table of Contents

Introduction

You will not get an exact definition of the word "diabetes" because there is more than one type. For example, there is Diabetes Insipidus, a condition characterized by heightened thirst and dilute urine. Pre-diabetes is a condition where your blood sugar level tends to be higher than usual after fasting - the medical term is impaired fasting glucose. The sugar level can also be higher after eating - the medical term is impaired glucose tolerance. Gestational diabetes refers to the type that can occur during pregnancy.

However, when most people say "diabetes", they are likely to be referring to Type-2 Diabetes, which is the condition typified by a high blood sugar level. It is a metabolic condition. The body does not produce the correct level of insulin, or expresses inappropriate response to the produced insulin, and causes the level of glucose in the blood to increase.

The Importance of Insulin The one common factor, in every type of diabetes, is the function of the hormone, insulin. It is responsible for how your body stores and uses the glucose obtained from the carbohydrates you eat.

The pancreas produces insulin, in what are called beta cells. These cells primary function is to store and release insulin into the bloodstream. The beta cells respond to an increase in the amount of glucose in the blood by secreting insulin.

Glucose is needed by the body, as it is can easily break it down for energy use. A person with low levels of glucose in their bloodstream may feel lethargic, dizzy, and their muscles may shake. However, a person with high amounts of glucose in their blood may experience blurred vision, a frequent urge to urinate, severe thirst, anxiety, muscle tingling, and fatigue.

Having an abnormally low or high level of glucose in your bloodstream is dangerous. Having a low amount of glucose may cause your body and brain to shut down; while too much glucose may be toxic.

A healthy body produces insulin to ensure there is just enough glucose in the bloodstream to function on any given day. The amount a person requires varies according to their daily physical activity. An athlete or a person that exercises regularly may need more glucose. A person who is not as active will need less glucose.

A diagnosis of diabetes can be frightening. You may be in a state of shock and vaguely hear your doctor talk about blood sugar numbers, blood testing, medications, and potential complications. For many people, their thoughts immediately turn to food. After all, eating is one of life's greatest pleasures. As a certified diabetes educator, the first questions my patients usually ask me are, "What can I eat? Will I have to cut out my favorite foods? Are bread, pasta, and sweets off-limits forever? How will I cook for my family if I have to be on a special diet?"

The changes you have to make might feel overwhelming. Conflicting advice from friends and the media can make things even more confusing. But here's the good news: Type 2 diabetes is manageable. Best of all, you will still be able to eat your favorite foods. And yes, that does include bread, pasta, and sweets — in moderation, of course! The Type 2 Diabetic Cookbook and Action Plan is here to help you. We will give you step-by-step guidance on tackling the diet and lifestyle changes that can help you manage type 2 diabetes. So . . . take a deep breath and read on.

The main goal of type 2 diabetes treatment is to effectively manage your blood sugar through food choices and physical activity. Good blood sugar control is important in order to help prevent complications. While some people may need medications, the good news is that many people can manage their diabetes with lifestyle changes alone. That includes losing weight if you are overweight, exercising regularly, and eating a healthy diet.

In the past, diabetic diets were very restrictive. Thirty years ago, when I first started counseling patients with diabetes, I remember advising them to avoid sugar and all desserts and to follow a rigid "exchange" type plan. Food was divided into six different groups, or exchange lists. Each exchange list contained foods with about the same amount of carbohydrate, protein, fat, and calories. For example, for breakfast you might be allowed one fruit exchange, two bread exchanges, one milk exchange, one meat exchange, and one fat exchange. While this system can be helpful for meal planning, it can also be somewhat inflexible.

But times have changed! While you will probably need to make some changes in what you are eating, you will have the flexibility to include the foods you enjoy. Adjusting to a new relationship with food can be challenging, and we're here for you every step of the way. We want to make it easy, so you don't feel overwhelmed. That's why we've taken the guesswork out of what to eat to manage your diabetes.

Recipes

Breakfast

1 Bulgur Porridge

Preparation time: 10 Minutes

Cooking time: 30 minutes

Servings: 2

Ingredients:

2/3 cup unsweetened soy milk

1/3 cup bulgur, rinsed

Pinch of salt

1 ripe banana, peeled and mashed

2 kiwis, peeled and sliced

Directions:

In a pan, add the soy milk, bulgur, and salt over medium-high heat and bring to a boil.

Adjust the heat to low and simmer for about 10 minutes.

Remove the pan of bulgur from heat and immediately, stir in the mashed banana.

Serve warm with the topping of kiwi slices.

Nutrition: Calories 223 Total Fat 2.3 g Saturated Fat 0.3 g Cholesterol 0 mg Sodium 126 mg Total Carbs 47.5 g Fiber 8.6 g Sugar 17.4 g Protein 7.1 g

2 Turkey-broccoli Brunch Casserole

Preparation time: 10 Minutes

Cooking time: 30 minutes

Servings: 6

Ingredients:

2-1/2 cups turkey breast, cubed and cooked

16 oz. broccoli, chopp ed and drained

1-1/2 cups of milk, fat-free

1 cup cheddar cheese, low-fat, shredded

10 oz. cream of chicken soup. low sodium and low fat

What you will need from the store cupboard:

8 oz. egg substitute

¼ teaspoon of poultry seasoning

¼ cup of sour cream, low fat

½ teaspoon pepper

1/8 teaspoon salt

2 cups of seasoned stuffing cubes

Cooking spray

Directions:

Bring together the egg substitute, soup, milk, pepper, sour cream, salt, and poultry seasoning in a big bowl.

Now stir in the broccoli, turkey, ¾ cup of cheese and stuffing cubes.

Transfer to a baking dish. Apply cooking spray.

Bake for 10 minutes. Sprinkle the remaining cheese.

Bake for another 5 minutes.

Keep it aside for 5 minutes. Serve.

Nutrition: Calories 303, Carbohydrates 26g, Fiber 3g, Sugar 0.8g, Cholesterol 72mg, Total Fat 7g, Protein 33g

3 Cheesy Low-carb Omelet

Preparation time: 10 Minutes

Cooking time: 30 minutes

Servings: 5

Ingredients:

2 whole eggs

1 tablespoon water

1 tablespoon butter

3 thin slices salami

5 fresh basil leaves

5 thin slices, fresh ripe tomatoes

2 ounces fresh mozzarella cheese

Salt and pepper as needed

Directions:

Take a small bowl and whisk in eggs and water

Take a nonstick Sauté pan and place it over medium heat, add butter and let it melt

Pour egg mixture and cook for 30 seconds

Spread salami slices on half of egg mix and top with cheese, tomatoes, basil slices

Season with salt and pepper according to your taste

Cook for 2 minutes and fold the egg with the empty half

Cover and cook on LOW for 1 minute

Serve and enjoy!

Nutrition: Calories: 451; Fat: 36gCarbohydrates: 3gProtein:33g

4 Apple & Cinnamon Pancake

Preparation time: 10 Minutes

Cooking time: 30 minutes

Servings: 4

Ingredients:

¼ teaspoon ground cinnamon

1 ¾ cups Better Baking Mix

1 tablespoon oil

1 cup water

2 egg whites

½ cup sugar-free applesauce

Cooking spray

1 cup plain yogurt

Sugar substitute

Directions:

Blend the cinnamon and the baking mix in a bowl.

Create a hole in the middle and add the oil, water, egg and applesauce.

Mix well.

Spray your pan with oil.

Place it on medium heat.

Pour ¼ cup of the batter.

Flip the pancake and cook until golden.

Serve with yogurt and sugar substitute.

Nutrition: Calories 231 Total Fat 6 g Saturated Fat 1 g Cholesterol 54 mg Sodium 545 mg Total Carbohydrate 37 g Dietary Fiber 4 g Total Sugars 1 g Protein 8 g Potassium 750 mg

5 Guacamole Turkey Burgers

Preparation time: 10 Minutes

Cooking time: 30 minutes

Servings: 3

Ingredients:

12 oz. turkey, ground

1-1/2 avocados

2 teaspoons of juice from a lime

½ teaspoon cumin

1 red chili, chopped

What you will need from the store cupboard:

½ teaspoon garlic powder

½ teaspoon onion powder

3 teaspoons of olive oil

½ teaspoon salt

Directions:

Mix the turkey with the cumin, chili, salt, garlic powder, and onion powder in a medium-sized bowl.

Create 3 patties

Pour 3 teaspoons olive oil in a skillet and heat over medium heat.

Now cook your patties. Make sure that both sides are brown. Make the guacamole in the meantime.

Mash together the garlic powder, juice from lime and avocados in a bowl.

Add salt for seasoning.

Serve the burgers with guacamole on the patties.

Nutrition: Calories 316, Carbohydrates 9g, Fiber 8g, Sugar 0g, Cholesterol 80mg, Total Fat 21g, Protein 24g

6 Ham and Goat Cheese Omelet

Preparation time: 10 Minutes

Cooking time: 30 minutes

Servings: 1

Ingredients:

1 slice of ham, chopped

4 egg whites

2 teaspoons of water

2 tablespoons onion, chopped

1 tablespoon parsley, minced

What you will need from the store cupboard:

2 tablespoons green pepper, chopped

1/8 teaspoon pepper

2 tablespoons goat cheese, crumbled

Cooking spray

Directions:

Whisk together the water, pepper and egg whites in a bowl till everything blends well.

Stir in the green pepper, ham, and onion.

Now heat your skillet over medium heat after applying the cooking spray.

Pour in the egg white mix towards the edge.

As it sets, push the cooked parts to the center. Allow the uncooked portions to flow underneath.

Sprinkle the goat cheese to one side when there is no liquid egg.

Now fold your omelet into half.

Sprinkle the parsley.

Nutrition: Calories 143, Carbohydrates 5g, Fiber 1g, Sugar 0.3g, Cholesterol 27mg, Total Fat 4g, Protein 21g

7 Cloud Bread

Preparation Time: 10 Minutes

Cooking Time: 15 Minutes

Servings: 10

Ingredients:

4 Eggs, large & separated

½ tsp. Garlic Powder

½ tsp. Cream of Tartar

½ tsp. Sea Salt

2 oz. Cream Cheese, low-fat

1 tsp. Italian Seasoning

Directions:

Preheat the oven to 300° F.

Next, keep the egg whites in a large mixing bowl and to this, spoon in the cream of tartar.

Whip it on high power until it turns to soft meringue peaks. Transfer to another bowl.

Place the cream of cheese into the large bowl and whip on high power to soften.

Stir in the egg one by one into the mixture and whisk it well each time before adding each egg. Repeat the procedure until the whole mixture becomes smooth.

Spoon in the Italian seasoning, salt, and garlic powder.

Gently fold the egg white to the mixture while maintaining the foamy texture.

Take ¼ cup portion of the mixture to the greased baking sheet and spread to 4-inch circles. Leave ample space between each.

Finally, bake them for 15 to 20 minutes or until they golden on the outside and firm inside.

Cool for several minutes and then serve.

Tip: You can reduce the amount of garlic powder if desired.

Nutrition: Calories: 36Kcal Carbohydrates: 1g Proteins: 2g Fat: 2g Sodium: 167mg

Grains

8 Lentil And Chickpea Curry

Preparation time: 10 minutes

Cooking time: 30 minutes

Servings: 2

Ingredients:

2 cups dry lentils and chickpeas

1 thinly sliced onion

1 cup chopped tomato

3 tbsps. curry paste

1 tbsp. oil or ghee

Directions:

Set the Instant Pot to sauté and add the onion, oil, and curry paste.

When the onion is soft, add the remaining ingredients and seal.

Cook on Stew for 20 minutes.

Release the pressure naturally and serve.

Nutrition: Calories 360, Carbs 26g, Fat 19g, Protein 23g, Potassium (K) 866.5 mg, Sodium (Na) 964.4mg

9 Lentil And Eggplant Stew

Preparation time: 10 minutes

Cooking time: 30 minutes

Servings: 2

Ingredients:

1 lb. eggplant

1 lb. dry lentils

1 cup chopped vegetables

1 cup low sodium vegetable broth

Directions:

Mix all the ingredients in your Instant Pot, cook on Stew for 35 minutes.

Release the pressure naturally and serve.

Nutrition: Calories 310, Carbs 22g, Fat 10g, Protein 32g, Potassium (K) 670.6 mg, Sodium (Na) 267 mg

10   Eggplant Curry

Preparation time: 10 minutes

Cooking time: 30 minutes

Servings: 2

Ingredients:

2-3 cups chopped eggplant

1 thinly sliced onion

1 cup coconut milk

3tbsp curry paste

1tbsp oil or ghee

Directions:

Set the Instant Pot to saute and add the onion, oil, and curry paste.

When the onion is soft, add the remaining ingredients and seal.

Cook on Stew for 20 minutes. Release the pressure naturally.

Nutrition: Calories: 350;Carbs: 15 ;Sugar: 3 ;Fat: 25 ;Protein: 11 ;GL: 10

11   Pea And Mint Soup

Preparation time: 10 minutes

Cooking time: 30 minutes

Servings: 2

Ingredients:

1lb green peas

2 cups low sodium vegetable broth

3tbsp mint sauce

Directions:

Mix all the ingredients in your Instant Pot.

Cook on Stew for 35 minutes.

Release the pressure naturally.

Blend into a rough soup.

Nutrition: Calories: 130;Carbs: 17 ;Sugar: 4 ;Fat: 5 ;Protein: 19 ;GL: 11

12   Steamed Asparagus

Preparation time: 10 minutes

Cooking time: 30 minutes

Servings: 4

Ingredients:

1 lb. fresh asparagus, rinsed and tough ends trimmed

1 cup water

Directions:

Place the asparagus into a wire steamer rack, and set it inside your Instant Pot.

Add water to the pot. Close and seal the lid, turning the steam release valve to the "Sealing" position.

Select the "Steam" function to cook on high pressure for 2 minutes.

Once done, do a quick pressure release of the steam.

Lift the wire steamer basket out of the pot and place the asparagus onto a serving plate.

Season as desired and serve.

Nutrition: Calories 22, Carbs 4g, Fat 0 g, Protein 2g, Potassium (K) 229 mg, Sodium (Na) 5 mg

---

Seafood

13   Crab Curry

Preparation time: 10 minutes

Cooking time: 30 minutes

Servings: 2

Ingredients:

0.5lb chopped crab

1 thinly sliced red onion

0.5 cup chopped tomato

3tbsp curry paste

1tbsp oil or ghee

Directions:

Set the Instant Pot to sauté and add the onion, oil, and curry paste.

When the onion is soft, add the remaining ingredients and seal.

Cook on Stew for 20 minutes.

Release the pressure naturally.

Nutrition: Calories 2; Carbs 11; Sugar 4; Fat 10; Protein 24; GL 9

14   Mussels in Tomato Sauce

Preparation time: 10 minutes

Cooking time: 30 minutes

Servings: 4

Ingredients:

2 tomatoes, seeded and chopped finely

2 pounds mussels, scrubbed and de-bearded

1 cup low-sodium chicken broth

1 tablespoon fresh lemon juice

2 garlic cloves, minced

Directions:

In the pot of Instant Pot, place tomatoes, garlic, wine and bay leaf and stir to combine.

Arrange the mussels on top.

Close the lid and place the pressure valve to "Seal" position.

Press "Manual" and cook under "High Pressure" for about 3 minutes.

Press "Cancel" and carefully allow a "Quick" release.

Open the lid and serve hot.

Nutrition: Calories 213, Fats 25.2g, Carbs 11g, Sugar 1. Proteins 28.2g, Sodium 670mg

15   Shrimp Salad

Preparation time: 10 minutes

Cooking time: 30 minutes

Servings: 6

Ingredients:

For Salad:

1 pound shrimp, peeled and deveined

Salt and ground black pepper, as required

1 teaspoon olive oil

1½ cups carrots, peeled and julienned

1½ cups red cabbage, shredded

1½ cup cucumber, julienned

5 cups fresh baby arugula

¼ cup fresh basil, chopped

¼ cup fresh cilantro, chopped

4 cups lettuce, torn

¼ cup almonds, chopped

For Dressing:

2 tablespoons natural almond butter

1 garlic clove, crushed

1 tablespoon fresh cilantro, chopped

1 tablespoon fresh lime juice

1 tablespoon unsweetened applesauce

2 teaspoons balsamic vinegar

½ teaspoon cayenne pepper

Salt, as required

1 tablespoon water

1/3 cup olive oil

Directions:

Slowly, add the oil, beating continuously until smooth.

For salad: in a bowl, add shrimp, salt, black pepper and oil and toss to coat well.

Heat a skillet over medium-high heat and cook the shrimp for about 2 minutes per side.

Remove from the heat and set aside to cool.

In a large bowl, add the shrimp, vegetables and mix well.

For dressing: in a bowl, add all ingredients except oil and beat until well combined.

Place the dressing over shrimp mixture and gently, toss to coat well.

Serve immediately.

Meal Prep Tip: Divide dressing in 6 large mason jars evenly. Place the remaining ingredients in the layers of carrots, followed by cabbage, cucumber, arugula, basil, cilantro, shrimp, lettuce and almonds. Cover each jar with the lid tightly and refrigerate for about 1 day. Shake the jars well just before serving.

Nutrition: Calories 274 Total Fat 17.7 g Saturated Fat 2.4 g Cholesterol 159 mg Total Carbs 10 g Sugar 3.8 g Fiber 2.9 g Sodium 242 mg Potassium 481 mg Protein 20.5 g

16 Grilled Herbed Salmon With Raspberry Sauc e & Cuc umber Dill Dip

Preparation time: 10 minutes

Cooking time: 30 minutes

Servings: 4

Ingredients:

3 salmon fillets

1 tablespoon olive oil

Salt and pepper to taste

1 teaspoon fresh sage, chopped

1 tablespoon fresh parsley, chopped

2 tablespoons apple juice

1 cup raspberries

1 teaspoon Worcestershire sauce

1 cup cucumber, chopped

2 tablespoons light mayonnaise

½ teaspoon dried dill

Directions:

Coat the salmon fillets with oil.

Season with salt, pepper, sage and parsley.

Cover the salmon with foil.

Grill for 20 minutes or until fish is flaky.

While waiting, mix the apple juice, raspberries and Worcestershire sauce.

Pour the mixture into a saucepan over medium heat.

Bring to a boil and then simmer for 8 minutes.

In another bowl, mix the rest of the ingredients.

Serve salmon with raspberry sauce and cucumber dip.

Nutrition: Calories 301 Fat 27.2 g Carbohydrates 13.6 g Protein 4.9 g Cholesterol 33 mg

17   Cajun Shrimp & Roasted Vegetables

Preparation time: 10 minutes

Cooking time: 30 minutes

Servings: 4

Ingredients:

1 lb. large shrimp, peeled and deveined

2 zucchinis, sliced

2 yellow squash, sliced

½ bunch asparagus, cut into thirds

2 red bell pepper, cut into chunks

What you'll need from store cupboard:

2 tbsp. olive oil

2 tbsp. Cajun Seasoning

Salt & pepper, to taste

Directions:

Heat oven to 400 degrees.

Combine shrimp and vegetables in a large bowl. Add oil and seasoning and toss to coat.

Spread evenly in a large baking sheet and bake 15-20 minutes, or until vegetables are tender. Serve.

Nutrition: Calories 251 Total Carbs 13g Net Carbs 9g Protein 30g Fat 9g Sugar 6g Fiber 4g

---

Poultry

18   Jerk Style Chicken Wings

Preparation time: 10 minutes

Cooking time: 30 minutes

Servings: 2-3

Ingredients:

1g ground thyme

1g dried rosemary

2g allspice

4g ground ginger

3 g garlic powder

2g onion powder

1g of cinnamon

2g of paprika

2g chili powder

1g nutmeg

Salt to taste

30 ml of vegetable oil

0.5 - 1 kg of chicken wings

1 lime, juice

Directions:

Select Preheat, set the temperature to 200°C and press Start/Pause.

Combine all spices and oil in a bowl to create a marinade.

Mix the chicken wings in the marinade until they are well covered.

Place the chicken wings in the preheated air fryer.

Select Chicken and press Start/Pause. Be sure to shake the baskets in the middle of cooking.

Remove the wings and place them on a serving plate.

Squeeze fresh lemon juice over the wings and serve.

Nutrition: Calories: 240 Fat: 15g Carbohydrate: 5g Protein: 19g Sugars: 4g Cholesterol: 60mg

19   Italian Chicken

Preparation time: 10 minutes

Cooking time: 30 minutes

Servings: 4

Ingredients:

5 chicken thighs

1 tbsp. olive oil

1/4 cup parmesan; grated

1/2 cup sun dried tomatoes

2 garlic cloves; minced

1 tbsp. thyme; chopped.

1/2 cup heavy cream

3/4 cup chicken stock

1 tsp. red pepper flakes; crushed

2 tbsp. basil; chopped

Salt and black pepper to the taste

Directions:

Season chicken with salt and pepper, rub with half of the oil, place in your preheated air fryer at 350 °F and cook for 4 minutes.

Meanwhile; heat up a pan with the rest of the oil over medium high heat, add thyme garlic, pepper flakes, sun dried tomatoes, heavy cream, stock, parmesan, salt and pepper; stir, bring to a simmer, take off heat and transfer to a dish that fits your air fryer.

Add chicken thighs on top, introduce in your air fryer and cook at 320 °F, for 12 minutes. Divide among plates and serve with basil sprinkled on top.

Nutrition: Calories: 272; Fat: 9; Fiber: 12; Carbs: 37; Protein: 23

20   Coconut Chicken

Preparation time: 10 minutes

Cooking time: 30 minutes

Servings: 6

Ingredients:

2 garlic cloves, minced

Fresh cilantro, minced

1/2 cup light coconut milk

6 tablespoons sweetened coconut, shredded and toasted

2 tablespoons brown sugar

6 (about 1-1/2 pounds) boneless skinless chicken thighs

2 tablespoons reduced-sodium soy sauce

1/8 teaspoon ground cloves

Directions:

Mix brown sugar, 1/2 cup light coconut milk, 2 tablespoons soy sauce, 1/8 teaspoon ground cloves and 2 minced cloves of garlic in a bowl.

Add 6 chicken boneless thighs into a Crockpot.

Now pour the mixture of coconut milk over chicken thighs.

Cover the cooker and cook for about 4-5 hours on low.

Serve coconut chicken with cilantro and coconut; enjoy!

Nutrition: 201 calories; 10 g fat; 6 g total carbs; 21 g protein

21   Spicy Lime Chicken

Preparation time: 10 minutes

Cooking time: 30 minutes

Servings: 6

Ingredients:

3 tablespoons lime juice

Fresh cilantro leaves

1-1/2 pounds (about 4) boneless skinless chicken breast halves

1 teaspoon lime zest, grated

2 cups chicken broth

1 tablespoon chili powder

Directions:

Add chicken breast halves into a slow cooker.

Add 1 tablespoon chili powder, 3 tablespoons lime juice and 2 cups chicken broth in a small bowl; mix well and pour over chicken.

Cover the cooker and cook for about 3 hours on low. Once done, take chicken out from the cooker and let it cool.

Once cooled, shred chicken by using forks and transfer back to the Crockpot.

Stir in 1 teaspoon grated lime zest. Serve spicy lime chicken with cilantro and enjoy!

Nutrition: 132 calories; 3 g fat; 2 g total carbs; 23 g protein

Preparation time: 10 minutes

Cooking time: 30 minutes

Servings: 4

Ingredients:

1 cup chive and onion cream cheese spread

½ teaspoon freshly ground black pepper

4 boneless chicken breasts

1 1-oz package ranch dressing and seasoning mix

½ cup low sodium chicken stock

Directions:

Spray the Crock-Pot slow cooker with cooking spray and preheat it.

Dry chicken with paper towel and transfer it to the Crock-Pot slow cooker.

Cook each side, until chicken is browned, for about 4-5 minutes.

Add ½ cup low sodium chicken stock, 1 1-oz. package ranch dressing and seasoning mix, 1 cup chive and onion cream cheese spread and ½ teaspoon freshly ground black pepper.

Cover the Crock-Pot slow cooker and cook for about 4 hours on Low or until the internal temperature reaches 165 F. Once cooked, take it out from the Crock-Pot slow cooker.

Whisk the sauce present in the Crock-Pot slow cooker until smooth. If you need thick sauce, then cook for about 5-10 minutes, with frequent stirring.

Garnish chicken with sliced onions and bacon and serve.

Nutrition: 362 calories; 18.5 g fat; 9.7 g total carbs; 37.3 g protein

23   Chicken Wings

Preparation time: 10 Minutes

Cooking time: 1 hour and 30 minutes

Servings: 4

Ingredients:

3 pounds chicken wing parts, pastured

1 tablespoon old bay seasoning

1 teaspoon lemon zest

3/4 cup potato starch

1/2 cup butter, unsalted, melted

Directions:

Switch on the air fryer, insert fryer basket, grease it with olive oil, then shut with its lid, set the fryer at 360 degrees F and preheat for 5 minutes.

Meanwhile, pat dry chicken wings and then place them in a bowl.

Stir together seasoning and starch, add to chicken wings and stir well until evenly coated.

Open the fryer, add chicken wings in it in a single layer, close with its lid and cook for 35 minutes, shaking every 10 minutes. Then switch the temperature of air fryer to 400 degrees F and continue air frying the chicken wings for 10 minutes or until nicely golden brown and cooked, shaking every 3 minutes. When air fryer beeps, open its lid, transfer chicken wings onto a serving plate and cook the remaining wings in the same manner.

Whisk together melted butter and lemon zest until blended and serve it with the chicken wings.

Nutrition:

Calories: 240 Cal

Carbs: 4 g

Fat: 16 g

Protein: 20 g

Fiber: 0 g

Soup and Stews

24   Zucchini Soup

Preparation time: 10 minutes

Cooking time: 30 minutes

Servings: 2

Ingredients:

2 medium zucchinis, chopped

1/2 teaspoon onion powder

1/2 teaspoon garlic powder

1/2 teaspoon salt

1/4 teaspoon ground black pepper

1/2 teaspoon curry powder

1 cup coconut milk, reduced-fat and unsweetened

1 cup of water

Directions:

Plugin instant pot, insert the inner pot, pour in water, then insert steamer basket and place zucchini pies on it.

Shut the instant pot with its lid and turn the pressure knob to seal the pot.

Press the 'steam' button, then press the 'timer' to set the cooking time to 2 minutes and cook at high pressure, instant pot will take 5 minutes or more for building its inner pressure.

When the timer beeps, press 'cancel' button and do natural pressure release for 5 minutes and then do quick pressure release until pressure nob drops down.

Open the instant pot, transfer zucchini to a plate to cool for 5 minutes, then place zucchini pieces in a food processor and add remaining ingredients.

Pulse zucchini for 1 to 2 minutes or until smooth and then evenly divide between bowls.

Serve straight away.

Nutrition: Calories: 141 Cal, Carbs: 7 g, Fat: 11 g, Protein: 3.5 g, Fiber: 3 g.

25   French Onion Soup

Preparation time: 10 minutes

Cooking time: 30 minutes

Servings: 2

Ingredients:

6 onions, chopped finely

2 cups vegetable broth

2tbsp oil

2tbsp Gruyere

Directions:

Place the oil in your Instant Pot and cook the onions on Saute until soft and brown.

Mix all the ingredients in your Instant Pot.

Cook on Stew for 35 minutes.

Release the pressure naturally.

Nutrition: Calories: 110;Carbs: 8 ;Sugar: 3 ;Fat: 10 ;Protein: 3 ;GL: 4

26   Beansprout Soup

Preparation time: 10 minutes

Cooking time: 30 minutes

Servings: 2

Ingredients:

1 lb. beansprouts

1 lb. chopped vegetables

1 cup low sodium broth

1 tbsp. mixed herbs

1 minced onion

Directions:

Mix all the ingredients in your Instant Pot, cook on Stew for 10 minutes.

Release the pressure naturally and serve.

Nutrition: Calories 100, Carbs 4g, Fat 10g, Protein 4g, Potassium (K) 349.9 mg, Sodium (Na) 310 mg

27   Shiitake Soup

Preparation time: 10 minutes

Cooking time: 30 minutes

Servings: 2

Ingredients:

1 cup shiitake mushrooms

1 cup diced vegetables

1 cup low sodium vegetable broth

2tbsp 5 spice seasoning

Directions:

Mix all the ingredients in your Instant Pot.

Cook on Stew for 35 minutes.

Release the pressure naturally.

Nutrition: Calories: 70;Carbs: 5 ;Sugar: 1 ;Fat: 2 ;Protein: 2 ;GL: 1

28   Pumpkin Soup

Preparation time: 10 minutes

Cooking time: 30 minutes

Servings: 2

Ingredients:

1 lb. chopped pumpkin

1 lb. chopped tomato

1 cup broth

1tbsp. mixed herbs

1 minced onion

Directions:

Mix all the ingredients in your Instant Pot.

Cook on Stew for 10 minutes.

Release the pressure naturally.

Blend.

Nutrition: Calories 200, Carbs 7g, Fat 11g, Protein 2g, Potassium (K) 259 mg, Sodium (Na) 1033 mg

29   Taco Soup

Preparation time: 10 minutes

Cooking time: 30 minutes

Servings: 4

Ingredients:

1 tbsp. olive oil

1 diced yellow onion

2 minced garlic cloves

15 oz. drained black beans

14 oz. crushed tomatoes

1 cup frozen sweetcorn

3 diced bell peppers

6 cups vegetable broth

1 box chickpea pasta shells

1 sliced jalapeño pepper, sliced

1 tbsp. chili powder

1 tsp. ground cuminutes

1 tsp. dried oregano

½ tsp. sea salt

To Serve:

Fresh cilantro

1 sliced avocado

Directions:

Add the olive oil, onions, garlic, tomatoes, corn, beans, spices and vegetable broth to Instant Pot. Stir gently.

Cover and seal the lid, making sure the steam release valve is set to "Sealing."

Cook on the "Manual, High Pressure" setting for 3 minutes, and once done, do a quick release of the pressure.

Stir in the diced bell peppers and chickpeas pasta, and then sit for 5-10 minutes.

Ladle the soup into bowls, top with the diced jalapeño, fresh cilantro and sliced avocados, and then serve.

Nutrition: Calories 430, Carbs 74g, Fat 9g, Protein 27g, Potassium (K) 620 mg, Sodium (Na) 921 mg

30   Vegetable Lentil Soup

Preparation time: 10 minutes

Cooking time: 30 minutes

Servings: 10

Ingredients:

1/4 cup soy protein

1/2 cup dried lentils, rinsed

1 large potato, peeled and diced

1 cup chopped carrots

1/2 cups diced green beans

1 cup chopped zucchini

1 medium tomato, chopped

1/2 cup diced white onion

1 teaspoon minced garlic

1 teaspoon salt

1/4 teaspoon ground black pepper

2 basil leaves

1/4 cup tomato sauce

4 cups vegetable stock

Directions:

Plugin instant pot, insert the inner pot, add all the ingredients, and stir until mixed.

Shut the instant pot with its lid and turn the pressure knob to seal the pot.

Press the 'slow cook' button, then press the 'timer' to set the cooking time to 6 hours at low heat setting.

When the timer beeps, press 'cancel' button and do natural pressure release for 10 minutes and then do quick pressure release until pressure nob drops down.

Open the instant pot, then ladle soup into bowls and serve.

Nutrition: Calories: 48.2 Cal, Carbs: 8.9 g, Fat: 0.2 g, Protein: 3.3 g, Fiber: 2.6 g.

31   Tofu Soup

Preparation time: 10 minutes

Cooking time: 30 minutes

Servings: 8

Ingredients:

1 lb. cubed extra-firm tofu

3 diced medium carrots

8 c. low-sodium vegetable broth

½ tsp. freshly ground white pepper

8 minced garlic cloves

6 sliced and divided scallions

4 oz. sliced mushrooms

1-inch minced fresh ginger piece

Directions:

Pour the broth into a stockpot. Add all of the ingredients except for the tofu and last 2 scallions. Bring to a boil over high heat.

Once boiling, add the tofu. Reduce heat to low, cover, and simmer for 5 minutes.

Remove from heat, ladle soup into bowls, and garnish with the remaining sliced scallions. Serve immediately.

Nutrition: Calories: 91, Fat:3 g, Carbs:8 g, Protein:6 g, Sugars:4 g, Sodium:900 mg

Salads, Sauces, Dressings & Dips

32   Tarragon Spring Peas

Preparation Time: 10 minutes

Cooking Time: 12 minutes

Serving: 6

Ingredients:

1 tablespoon unsalted butter

½ Vidalia onion

1 cup low-sodium vegetable broth

3 cups fresh shelled peas

1 tablespoon minced fresh tarragon

Directions:

Cook butter in a pan at medium heat.

Sauté the onion in the melted butter for about 3 minutes, stirring occasionally.

Pour in the vegetable broth and whisk well. Add the peas and tarragon to the skillet and stir to combine.

Reduce the heat to low, cover, cook for about 8 minutes more, or until the peas are tender.

Let the peas cool for 5 minutes and serve warm.

Nutrition:

82 calories

12g carbohydrates

3.8g fiber

33   Butter-Orange Yams

Preparation Time: 7 minutes

Cooking Time: 45 minutes

Serving: 8

Ingredients:

2 medium jewel yams

2 tablespoons unsalted butter

Juice of 1 large orange

1½ teaspoons ground cinnamon

¼ teaspoon ground ginger

¾ teaspoon ground nutmeg

1/8 teaspoon ground cloves

Directions:

Set oven at 180ºC.

Arrange the yam dices on a rimmed baking sheet in a single layer. Set aside.

Add the butter, orange juice, cinnamon, ginger, nutmeg, and garlic cloves to a medium saucepan over medium-low heat. Cook for 3 to 5 minutes, stirring continuously.

Spoon the sauce over the yams and toss to coat well.

Bake in the prepared oven for 40 minutes.

Let the yams cool for 8 minutes on the baking sheet before removing and serving.

Nutrition:

129 calories

24.7g carbohydrates

5g fiber

34 Roasted Tomato Brussels Sprouts

Preparation Time: 15 minutes

Cooking Time: 20 minutes

Serving: 4

Ingredients:

1-pound (454 g) Brussels sprouts

1 tablespoon extra-virgin olive oil

½ cup sun-dried tomatoes

2 tablespoons lemon juice

1 teaspoon lemon zest

Directions:

Set oven 205°C. Prep large baking sheet with aluminum foil.

Toss the Brussels sprouts in the olive oil in a large bowl until well coated. Sprinkle with salt and pepper.

Spread out the seasoned Brussels sprouts on the prepared baking sheet in a single layer.

Roast for 20 minutes, shake halfway through.

Remove from the oven then situate in a bowl. Whisk tomatoes, lemon juice, and lemon zest, to incorporate. Serve immediately.

Nutrition:

111 calories

13.7g carbohydrates

4.9g fiber

35   Simple Sautéed Greens

Preparation Time: 10 minutes

Cooking Time: 10 minutes

Serving: 4

Ingredients:

2 tablespoons extra-virgin olive oil

1 pound (454 g) Swiss chard

1-pound (454 g) kale

½ teaspoon ground cardamom

1 tablespoon lemon juice

Directions:

Heat up olive oil in a big skillet over medium-high heat.

Stir in Swiss chard, kale, cardamom, lemon juice to the skillet, and stir to combine. Cook for about 10 minutes, stirring continuously, or until the greens are wilted.

Sprinkle with the salt and pepper and stir well.

Serve the greens on a plate while warm.

Nutrition:

139 calories

15.8g carbohydrates

3.9g fiber

Dessert and Snacks

36   Fruit Kebab

Preparation time: 10 minutes

Cooking time: 30 minutes

Servings: 12

Ingredients:

3 apples

¼ cup orange juice

1 ½ lb. watermelon

¾ cup blueberries

Directions:

Use a star-shaped cookie cutter to cut out stars from the apple and watermelon.

Soak the apple stars in orange juice.

Thread the apple stars, watermelon stars and blueberries into skewers.

Refrigerate for 30 minutes before serving.

Nutrition: Calories 52 Total Fat 0 g Saturated Fat 0 g Cholesterol 0 mg Sodium 1 mg Total Carbohydrate 14 g Dietary Fiber 2 g Total Sugars 10 g Protein 1 g Potassium 134 mg

37 Cheese Berry Fat Bomb

Preparation time: 10 minutes

Cooking time: 30 minutes

Servings: 12

Ingredients:

1 cup fresh berries, wash

1/2 cup coconut oil

1 1/2 cup cream cheese, softened

1 tbsp vanilla

2 tbsp swerve

Directions:

Add all ingredients to the blender and blend until smooth and combined.

Spoon mixture into small candy molds and refrigerate until set.

Serve and enjoy.

Nutrition: Calories 175 Fat 17 g Carbohydrates 2 g Sugar 1 g Protein 2.1 g Cholesterol 29 mg

38 Tamari Toasted Almonds

Preparation time: 10 minutes

Cooking time: 30 minutes

Servings: ½

Ingredients:

½ cup raw almonds, or sunflower seeds

2 tablespoons tamari, or soy sauce

1 teaspoon toasted sesame oil

Directions:

Preparing the Ingredients

Heat a dry skillet to medium-high heat, then add the almonds, stirring frequently to keep them from burning. Once the almonds are toasted — 7-8 minutes for almonds, or 34 minutes for sunflower seeds — pour the tamari and sesame oil into the hot skillet and stir to coat.

You can turn off the heat, and as the almonds cool the tamari mixture will stick and dry on to the nuts.

Nutrition: Calories: 89 Total fat: 8g Carbs: 3g Fiber: 2g Protein: 4g

39   Choco Peppermint Cake

Preparation time: 10 minutes

Cooking time: 30 minutes

Servings: 4

Ingredients:

Cooking spray

⅓ cup oil

15 oz. package chocolate cake mix

3 eggs, beaten

1 cup water

¼ teaspoon peppermint extract

Directions:

Spray slow cooker with oil.

Mix all the ingredients in a bowl.

Use an electric mixer on medium speed setting to mix ingredients for 2 minutes.

Pour mixture into the slow cooker.

Cover the pot and cook on low for 3 hours.

Let cool before slicing and serving.

Nutrition: Calories 185 Total Fat 7.4 g Total Carbohydrate 27 g Protein 3.8 g

40   Frozen Lemon & Blueberry

Preparation time: 10 minutes

Cooking time: 30 minutes

Servings: 4

Ingredients:

6 cup fresh blueberries

8 sprigs fresh thyme

¾ cup light brown sugar

1 teaspoon lemon zest

¼ cup lemon juice

2 cups water

Directions:

Add blueberries, thyme and sugar in a pan over medium heat.

Cook for 6 to 8 minutes.

Transfer mixture to a blender.

Remove thyme sprigs.

Stir in the remaining ingredients.

Pulse until smooth.

Strain mixture and freeze for 1 hour.

Nutrition: Calories 78 Total Fat 0 g Total Carbohydrate 20 g Protein 3 g

41   Pumpkin & Banana Ice Cream

Preparation time: 10 minutes

Cooking time: 30 minutes

Servings: 4

Ingredients:

15 oz. pumpkin puree

4 bananas, sliced and frozen

1 teaspoon pumpkin pie spice

Chopped pecans

Directions:

Add pumpkin puree, bananas and pumpkin pie spice in a food processor.

Pulse until smooth.

Chill in the refrigerator.

Garnish with pecans.

Nutrition: Calories 71 Total Fat 0.4 g Total Carbohydrate 18 g Protein 1.2 g

42   Coconut Chia Pudding

Preparation time: 10 minutes

Cooking time: 0 minutes

Servings: 6

Ingredients:

2 ¼ cup canned coconut milk

1 teaspoon vanilla extract

Pinch salt

½ cup chia seeds

Directions:

Combine the coconut milk, vanilla, and salt in a bowl.

Stir well and sweeten with stevia to taste.

Whisk in the chia seeds and chill overnight.

Spoon into bowls and serve with chopped nuts or fruit.

Nutrition: 300 calories 27.5g fat 6g protein 14.5g carbs 10g fiber 4.5g net carbs

43   Strawberries In Honey Yogurt Dip

Preparation time: 10 minutes

Cooking time: 0 minutes

Servings: 4

Ingredients:

1 cup plain yogurt, low-fat

1 tablespoon of orange juice

1 to 2 teaspoons of honey

Ground cinnamon

1 quart of fresh strawberries (remove stems)

Directions:

Combine first four ingredients to make a sauce. Pour over strawberries and serve.

Nutrition: Calories: 88 Carbohydrates: 16 g Fiber: 4 g Fats: 1 g Sodium: 41 mg Protein: 4 g Diabetic Exchange: 1/2 Milk, 1 Fruit

44   Mortadella & Bacon Balls

Preparation time: 10 minutes

Cooking time: 30 minutes

Servings: 2

Ingredients:

4 ounces Mortadella sausage

4 bacon slices, cooked and crumbled

2 tbsp almonds, chopped

½ tsp Dijon mustard

3 ounces' cream cheese

Directions:

Combine the mortadella and almonds in the bowl of your food processor. Pulse until smooth. Whisk the cream cheese and mustard in another bowl. Make balls out of the mortadella mixture.

Make a thin cream cheese layer over. Coat with bacon, arrange on a plate and chill before serving.

Nutrition: Calories 547 Fat: 51g Net Carbs: 3.4g Protein: 21.5g

45   Tiramisu Shots

Preparation Time: 5 minutes

Cooking Time: 10 minutes

Servings: 4

Ingredients:

1 pack silken tofu

1 oz. dark chocolate, finely chopped

¼ cup sugar substitute

1 teaspoon lemon juice

¼ cup brewed espresso

Pinch salt

24 slices angel food cake

Cocoa powder (unsweetened)

Directions:

1. Add tofu, chocolate, sugar substitute, lemon juice, espresso and salt in a food processor.

2. Pulse until smooth.

3. Add angel food cake pieces into shot glasses.

4. Drizzle with the cocoa powder.

5. Pour the tofu mixture on top.

6. Top with the remaining angel food cake pieces.

7. Chill for 30 minutes and serve.

Nutrition:

75 Calories

12g Carbohydrate

2.9g Protein

46   Ice Cream Brownie Cake

Preparation Time: 5 minutes

Cooking Time: 10 minutes

Servings: 4

Ingredients:

Cooking spray

12 oz. no-sugar brownie mix

¼ cup oil

2 egg whites

3 tablespoons water

2 cups sugar-free ice cream

Directions:

1. Preheat your oven to 325 degrees F.

2. Spray your baking pan with oil.

3. Mix brownie mix, oil, egg whites and water in a bowl.

4. Pour into the baking pan.

5. Bake for 25 minutes.

6. Let cool.

7. Freeze brownie for 2 hours.

8. Spread ice cream over the brownie.

9. Freeze for 8 hours.

Nutrition:

198 Calories

33g Carbohydrate

3g Protein

47   Peanut Butter Cups

Preparation Time: 5 minutes

Cooking Time: 10 minutes

Servings: 4

Ingredients:

1 packet plain gelatin

¼ cup sugar substitute

2 cups nonfat cream

½ teaspoon vanilla

¼ cup low-fat peanut butter

2 tablespoons unsalted peanuts, chopped

Directions:

1. Mix gelatin, sugar substitute and cream in a pan.

2. Let sit for 5 minutes.

3. Place over medium heat and cook until gelatin has been dissolved.

4. Stir in vanilla and peanut butter.

5. Pour into custard cups. Chill for 3 hours.

6. Top with the peanuts and serve.

Nutrition:

171 Calories

21g Carbohydrate

6.8g Protein

48   Fruit Pizza

Preparation Time: 5 minutes

Cooking Time: 10 minutes

Servings: 4

Ingredients:

1 teaspoon maple syrup

¼ teaspoon vanilla extract

½ cup coconut milk yogurt

2 round slices watermelon

½ cup blackberries, sliced

½ cup strawberries, sliced

2 tablespoons coconut flakes (unsweetened)

Directions:

1. Mix maple syrup, vanilla and yogurt in a bowl.

2. Spread the mixture on top of the watermelon slice.

3. Top with the berries and coconut flakes.

Nutrition:

70 Calories

14.6g Carbohydrate

1.2g Protein

49   Choco Peppermint Cake

Preparation Time: 5 minutes

Cooking Time: 10 minutes

Servings: 4

Ingredients:

Cooking spray

1/3 cup oil

15 oz. package chocolate cake mix

3 eggs, beaten

1 cup water

¼ teaspoon peppermint extract

Directions:

1. Spray slow cooker with oil.

2. Mix all the ingredients in a bowl.

3. Use an electric mixer on medium speed setting to mix ingredients for 2 minutes.

4. Pour mixture into the slow cooker.

5. Cover the pot and cook on low for 3 hours.

6. Let cool before slicing and serving.

Nutrition:

185 Calories

27g Carbohydrate

3.8g Protein

50   Roasted Mango

Preparation Time: 5 minutes

Cooking Time: 10 minutes

Servings: 4

Ingredients:

2 mangoes, sliced

2 teaspoons crystallized ginger, chopped

2 teaspoons orange zest

2 tablespoons coconut flakes (unsweetened)

Directions:

1. Preheat your oven to 350 degrees F.

2. Add mango slices in custard cups.

3. Top with the ginger, orange zest and coconut flakes.

4. Bake in the oven for 10 minutes.

Nutrition:

89 Calories

20g Carbohydrate

0.8g Protein

Conclusion

I hope that this book was able to help you to fully understand the causes of Diabetes. I hope that this book was able to explain further the facts and information about Diabetes and I hope that by reading this book, you would soon be able to free yourself from Diabetes and become a healthier and happier person.

The next step is to use all of the new knowledge that you have earned from this book and to apply it on your lifestyle. The suggestions in this book that I have suggested will not only help you to cure or reduce Diabetes but also to save money from buying medicines. You can use the Action Plan to help you stop Diabetes in a more organized and strategically way. I wish you the best of luck!

Thank you and good luck!

Big thanks for purchasing this book and reading all the way to the end!

As earlier indicated, being diagnosed with diabetes is not a death sentence. With proper diet, exercise and a suitable lifestyle, you are well on your way to reversing diabetes.

Always remember that you have to start somewhere so even though it may seem difficult at the beginning, that it will get better with time and as you continue in consistency, you will feel better with each passing day until you feel new again and as though you have never had diabetes!

I hope this book has been of great help in providing you with the information you needed regarding being able to successfully manage diabetes symptoms as well as reversing the condition. Remember that it is never too late to start so start doing something now and enjoy the benefits.

CPSIA information can be obtained
at www.ICGtesting.com
Printed in the USA
BVHW041116010321
601386BV00009B/751

9 781801 654524